Dana Carpender's
Weight-Loss Tracker

Dana Carpender's
Weight-Loss Tracker

*A Daily Calorie, Carb, Protein, Fat,
and Exercise Journal
to Help You Lose Weight and Inches*

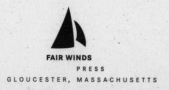

FAIR WINDS
PRESS
GLOUCESTER, MASSACHUSETTS

Text © 2005 by Dana Carpender

First published in the USA in 2005 by
Fair Winds Press
33 Commercial Street
Gloucester, MA 01930

08 07 06 05 04   1 2 3 4 5

ISBN 1-59233-151-3

Library of Congress Cataloging-in-Publication Data

Carpender, Dana.
  Dana Carpender's weight-loss tracker : a daily calorie, carb, protein, fat, and exercise journal
to help you lose weight and inches / Dana Carpender.
     p. cm.
  ISBN 1-59233-151-3
1. Weight loss. 2. Account books. I. Title: Weight-loss tracker. II. Title.
  RM222.2.C324 2005
  613.2'5--dc22
                                                                           2004023341

Cover design by Mary Ann Smith
Book design by Joanna Detz

Printed and bound in Canada

*The information in this book is for educational purposes only. It is not intended to replace the
advice of a physician or medical practitioner. Please see your health care provider before
beginning any new health program.*

Consciousness is
a very powerful tool.

CONTENTS

INTRODUCTION

I've been counting carbs for nine years, but I didn't always keep track, and that worked fine for me. However, age conspires against you. A woman's body retains fat in order to make up for the estrogen it loses from the ovaries. Men lose muscle-building testosterone as they age. So, you just can't eat the way you used to when you were young.

In my case, I was in a car accident and injured my right leg. I put some weight back on because I couldn't exercise. Finally, two years ago, I decided that being in pain wasn't as bad as being out of shape. I found a really good chiropractor, but there is still a limit to what kinds of exercise I can do. I do find that keeping track of everything really helps. The biggest way it helps is that it stops me from eating "unconsciously." I don't even have a rigid limit I stick to. Some days I go to 60 carbs and 2,200 calories and other days it's 25 carbs and 1,500 calories, but I always know what I've eaten.

By not eating "unconsciously" you force yourself to make better choices. This way, if you find yourself in the break room with the doughnuts, and say aloud to yourself: "Five minutes of eating doughnuts is worth three days of water weight gain and two hours of feeling lousy," then at least you've made a decision. And if you can say that happily, then knock yourself out.

How to Use This Journal

You need to write down everything, even if it's a food you wish you hadn't eaten. For example, the other day while dining out, I indulged in an ear of corn and a blooming onion. I went home and entered these foods into my journal, did some extra exercise, and then I watched what I ate the next day. I made better choices because I was conscious of what I had done.

So if you eat something bad, you must write it down. At the same time, if you eat something good, write it down.

Now, aside from writing down what food you're eating, you also have to write down how much of it you're eating. The notion that you can eat unlimited calories so long as you keep the carb count very low has been oversold. It does appear to be true that you can eat more calories on a low-carb diet than you could on a carb-rich diet and still lose weight, and you certainly never have to go hungry, but that doesn't mean you can eat 10,000 calories a day and still lose weight. To be true to yourself, your diet, and therefore your journal, you must take into account all factors—calories, carbs, fiber, protein, and fat.

Do yourself a favor and get in the habit of reading the label on every food product, and I do mean every food product, that has one. If you're in a position where you can't read the labels (for instance, at the deli counter at the grocery store), ask questions. The nice deli folks will be glad to read the labels on the ham and salami for you, and they can tell you what goes into the various items they make themselves. I've found that if I tell them I have a medical condition that requires me to be very careful about my diet—and I don't come at the busiest hour of the week—folks are generally very nice about this sort of thing.

I have learned from long, hard, repetitive experience that food manufacturers can, will, and do put sugar, corn syrup, corn starch, and other nutritionally empty, carb-laden garbage into every food product. I have found sugar in everything from salsa to canned clams, for heaven's sake! (Why clams need sugar, I'd love to know.) You will shave untold thousands of grams of carbs off your intake in the course of a year by simply looking for the product without the added junk.

There are a good many classes of food products out there to which sugar is virtually always added; the cured meats come to mind. There is almost always sugar in sausage, ham, bacon, hot dogs, liverwurst, and the like. You will look in vain for sugarless varieties of these products, which is one good reason why you should primarily eat fresh meats instead. However, you will find that there is quite a range of carb counts among cured meats, because some manufacturers add more sugar than others do. I have seen ham that has one gram of carbohydrate per serving, and I have seen ham that has six grams of carbohydrate per serving—that's a 600 percent difference! Likewise, I've seen hot dogs that have one gram of carbohydrate apiece, and I've seen hot dogs that have five grams of carbohydrate apiece. Be smart about your food choices, take time to do the research, and you will be rewarded.

In short, you need to become a food sleuth. After all, you're paying your hard-earned money for this stuff, and it is quite literally going to become a part of you. Pay at least as much attention as you would if you were buying a car or a computer.

How to Count a Serving

Packaged foods and my *Carb Gram Counter* tell you how big a serving is, but I've gotten a couple of queries from folks who bought *500 Low-Carb Recipes* and want to know how big a cookbook serving size is, so I thought I'd better address the matter.

To be quite honest, folks, there's no great technical determination going on here. For the most part, a "serving" is based on what I think would make a reasonabl portion, depending on the carbohydrate count, how rich the dish is, and, for main dishes, the protein count. You just divide up the dish into however many portions the recipe says, and trust that the carb counts for the recipes are accurate.

Of course, this "serving" thing is fluky. People are different sizes and have different appetites. For all I know, you have three children under five who might reasonably split one adult-size portion. On the other hand, you might have one seventeen-year-old boy who's shot up from 5'5" to 6'3" in the past year, and what looks like four servings to me will be a quick snack for him. You'll just have to eyeball what fraction of the whole dish you're eating, and go from there.

How to Count Carbs

It's important to know about "impact carbs," "usable carbs," "net carbs," or "effective carbs." These terms all refer to the grams of carbohydrate that you can actually digest and absorb. The carbohydrate chains that make up dietary fibers are just too big for the human gut to digest and absorb, which is why we can't live on grass like cows do. Accordingly, you can subtract the grams of fiber from the total grams of carbohydrate to get the number of grams of carbohydrate you actually need to worry about. This approach dramatically increases the amount of vegetables, fruits, nuts, seeds, and other plant foods you can eat.

Some other considerations to bear in mind:

- Beware of hidden carbohydrates. It's important to know that the government lets food manufacturers put "0 grams of carbohydrate" on the label if a food has less than 0.5 grams per serving, and "less than one gram of carbohydrate" if a food has between 0.5 grams and 0.9 grams. Even some diet sodas contain trace amounts of carbohydrates! These amounts aren't much, but they do add up if you eat enough of them. So if you're having trouble losing weight, count foods that say "0 grams" as 0.5 grams and foods that say "less than one gram" as one gram.

- Remember that some foods you may be thinking of as carb-free actually contain at least traces of carbohydrates. Eggs contain about 0.5 gram apiece, shrimp have one gram per four-ounce portion, natural cheeses have about one gram per ounce, and heavy cream has about 0.5 gram per tablespoon. Coffee has more than one gram in a ten-ounce mug *before* you add cream and sweetener. (Tea, on the other hand, is carb-free.) If you're having trouble losing weight, get a food counter book and use it, even for foods you're sure you already know the carb counts of.

- Do not make low-carb specialty products a major part of your diet. Low-carb breads, pastas, candy, cookies, protein bars, and so on, are flooding the market, and they do provide a nice variety. However, most of these products are not, as nutritious, healthful, or filling as real food. Furthermore, they're all extremely expensive! And almost all of them have more carbohydrates than a hard-boiled egg or a chicken wing. So stop trying to make your low-carb diet look like your old high-carb diet—that's the diet that got you in trouble in the first place, remember?

- Regarding those sugar-free chocolate bars, not to mention protein bars, jelly beans, brownies, and so on: Just about all of them are sweetened with polyols, sometimes called sugar alcohols. These are carbohydrates, but they're carbohydrates that are slowly and incompletely absorbed, at best. Because of this, all low-carb specialty food labels subtract out polyols from the total carb count, just like fiber. Polyol-sweetened treats are easier on your body than the sugar-sweetened kind, but it's optimistic to assume that none of that carbohydrate is absorbed. When low-carb sweets say you can subtract out *all* of the sugar alcohols from the carb count, take that with a grain of salt. Sugar alcohol is sometimes identified in labels as maltitol, which is said to be free of sugar, but I would say you should count half of that.

- Also be aware that polyols/sugar alcohols will cause gas and/or diarrhea if you eat them in any quantity. Be very careful with your portions. I rarely eat more than a half of a 1.5 ounce chocolate bar in a day. Don't eat sugar-free sweets at all before a big job interview, an important presentation, a hot date, or getting on a plane, or you may well be sorry.

- When you hit a plateau, lose the treats. The sugar-free chocolate bars and the low-carb baked goods are the first things to axe if you're not losing weight.

- Don't eat for entertainment! Eat when you're hungry, eat enough to feel satisfied, then quit until you're physically hungry again. It's a shame that we even need to be told this, it's so basic, but our society has developed a bad habit of eating for the fun of it, regardless of hunger.

- Don't be fooled by the fact that many alcoholic drinks have a low carb count. Alcohol in any form will slow fat-burning dramatically. This doesn't mean you can't drink at all, just realize that alcohol is *always* a major luxury on a weight-loss diet, and gauge your intake accordingly.

The heart and soul of your nutritional program, for the rest of your life, should be meat, fish, poultry, eggs, cheese, healthy fats, low-carb vegetables, low-sugar fruits, and nuts and seeds. You know— *food.* **A sugar-free candy bar or brownie or a bag of low-carb chips is** *never* **a substitute for a chicken Caesar salad for lunch. Got it?**

The Importance of Fiber

Fiber is a carbohydrate, and is, at least in American nutritional breakdowns, included in the total carbohydrate count. However, as I mentioned earlier, fiber is a form of carbohydrate made of molecules so big that you can neither digest nor absorb them. Therefore fiber, despite being a carbohydrate, will not push up your blood sugar and will not cause an insulin release. Even better, by slowing the absorption of the starches and sugars that occur with it, fiber actually lessens their bad influence. This is very likely the reason that high-fiber diets appear to be so much better for you than the "American Normal."

According to the government, you should try to eat at least twenty-five grams of fiber a day. I sometimes wonder if this is essential for low-carbers? People who eat a lot of refined sugar and starch need something to counteract that, but since low-carbers don't eat all of those refined foods, maybe the number can be lower. Fifteen grams of fiber a day might be a more realistic goal for most people.

The Importance of Water

Just as you need to be conscious about eating properly, you also need to be conscious about drinking properly. And that means making sure you get enough water. Eight glasses a day is the minimum that you should drink, and studies have now shown that at least some of this can be in the form of tea, coffee, or soda (as long as you aren't overdosing on caffeine!)

Basically, you know you're drinking enough water if your urine is fairly clear instead of bright yellow.

Make a note in your journal if you've had trouble making sure you're drinking enough water.

The Importance of Supplements

I recommend taking a multi-vitamin and a calcium/magnesium supplement every day, but I know a lot of people who are sure to take vitamin E for heart health and the B vitamins for stress relief and mood regulation. Whatever supplements you need, there is a place to enter them into this journal. Just fill it in. If you don't take anything, leave it blank.

However, if you're on a low-carb diet and are feeling tired as well as kind of achy, weak, or crampy, potassium loss—called "hypokalemia"—is likely to be your problem. And if this happens to you, get more potassium *right away*. Your heart needs potassium to run properly! *Don't mess around.* The best low-carb source of potassium is avocados; little black ones have eight grams of usable carbs apiece, and 1200 mgs of potassium. Green leafy vegetables are also a good low-carb source of potassium, as are fresh pork, fresh fish, cantaloupes, and almonds. Indeed, it's best to include these things in your diet from day one.

You can also take potassium tablets, if you like, but be aware that the doses tend to be low—just 99 mgs per tablet, when you need 2,000–3,000 mgs of potassium per day. Another way to supplement is to use Morton's Lite Salt, which combines the usual sodium-based salt with potassium-based salt. However, if you are on blood-pressure medication of any kind, check with your pharmacist or doctor before taking potassium supplements. Some blood pressure medications work by making your body hang on to potassium, and that makes it possible to get too much, which is as dangerous as too little.

Potassium imbalance is a temporary problem, caused by your body's shifting over from a high-carb diet, which makes you shed potassium and retain water, to a low-carb diet—which makes you dump all that excess water before your body stops shedding the potassium. Just include good potassium sources in your diet, and your body will sort it all out in a week or two.

The Importance of Exercise

Studies have shown that by beginning a regular strength-training practice, you can stave off a lot of the ravages of aging. It will also add muscle and speed your metabolism, making it far easier to control your weight.

You don't have to do strength training every day. I use a Total Gym every other day and it only takes about a half-hour to do the eight or so exercises you need to strengthen the major muscles of your body. There are lots of good workout books on the subject, such as *Tamilee Webb's Defy Gravity Workout*, but you can also hire a personal trainer to put you on a flexible program. You can find a good certified trainer at www.acsm.org.

The Importance of 10,000 Steps

Our lives have become ridiculously sedentary. Most of us don't even walk across the room to change the TV channel, so forget about walking downtown to shop or taking a walk to see our friends in the neighborhood. However, a person who walks 10,000 steps a day will burn between 2,000 and 3,500 extra calories per week, which will result in a vastly better health profile and longer lifespan.

Walking around 10,000 steps a day is equivalent to about five miles. The average person walks less than 6,000 steps per day. Many people need to include some type of daily walking program for about a half hour to one hour to get to 10,000 steps.

Investing in an inexpensive pedometer is a good way to begin and stay motivated with walking. Some pedometers can be adjusted to calculate miles, speed, and approximate calories burned, but simply monitoring the number of steps is enough and may be more accurate than some of the other measurements.

Determine your current number of steps for a couple of days and gradually build up. As a general guideline, a person will burn about 100 calories walking a mile. Fitness, weight, and age will affect how many calories each person burns.

If your goal is to lose weight, start slow and gradually work yourself up to walking 12,000 to 15,000 steps a day. Walking is a great way to lose weight—and keep it off.

Keeping Track of Your Weight

Don't become too obsessive about the scale because the scale is not the best way to gauge how fat you are. There are no magic answers here. Some people weigh themselves every day, some people lose weight by throwing out their scales. And some people use a favorite pair of jeans to gauge their weight rather than actually think about pounds—that's what I do.

I think this is all a matter of personal style, so I want you to know that you should feel free to ignore the spaces in this book that ask you to write down your weight or measurements. However, I did leave space in case you need it to keep yourself on track. It's up to you. The space is there, but it's not the most important part of this book. The most important part of this book is you—and your journey to becoming a conscious eater.

How Are You Doing?

Before you read further, ask yourself this question: "How am I doing?" Are you feeling hopeful because you're trying to get your eating on track? Or are you disappointed because you just binged or because you feel like you're out of shape? You may not believe this, but what's important about that question isn't the answer itself but how you answer it. If you're being honest and loving to yourself no matter what the answer, then you're on the right track.

In other words, even if you've just eaten half a fudge cake or even if you've just tried to get your size twelve jeans on and weren't able to zipper them, I want you to find a way to approve of yourself—and then set some sort of goal.

And, remember, a goal isn't a number, such as size four or 120 pounds. A goal is a plan; a workable, realistic plan that doesn't involve starvation. Instead, it should focus on something like eating enough low-carb vegetables or planning your meals around proteins rather than high-starch foods.

So, now when you answer the question "How am I doing?" I want you to be honest with yourself, nice to yourself, and if you don't like how you're doing, I want you to formulate a workable, realistic plan.

	Calories	Carbs	Fiber	Protein	Fat
Breakfast					
PORRIDGE	360	90	14	2	2
SUGAR	96	24	—	—	—
3 CUPS COFFEE	12	3	—	—	—
Lunch CHIPS	260	44	4	4	8
FISHCAKE	190	17	1	10	9
APPLE / BAN	80 110	49	2	1	1
3 BISCUITS	300	21	3	3	3
Dinner RICE	160	10			
CHEESE SAN	500	50			
APPLE / PEAR	130	34	8	2	1
1 BISCUIT	100	7	1	1	1
Snack					
2 FRUIT	190				
Snack					
2 FRUIT	150				
	2600	Burnt	3200 approx		

Did I reach my carb allowance with whole foods? (YES) NO	Did I get my minimum amount of protein today? (YES) NO

Low-carb vegetables

| Supplements : FISH OIL 100 G | Water |
| 1 COD LIVER OIL 100 G | |

| Exercise 85 MINS WEIGHTS 20 MINS CROSS TRAINER 1.30 1HR RUN 300.P.U. | 10,000 Steps |
| How I Did Today 5000   700 S.U. | Weight **81.5** |

1120 + 252 + 800 + 408 + ? 500 ?

	Calories	Carbs	Fiber	Protein	Fat
DATE			**DAY** MON. TUES. WED. THURS. FRI. SAT. SUN.		

	Calories	Carbs	Fiber	Protein	Fat
Breakfast					
Lunch					
Dinner					
Snack					
Snack					

Did I reach my carb
allowance with whole foods?   YES   NO

Did I get my minimum
amount of protein today?   YES   NO

Low-carb vegetables

Supplements

Water

Exercise

10,000 Steps

How I Did Today

Weight

DATE _____ **DAY**   MON.   TUES.   WED.   THURS.   FRI.   SAT.   SUN.

	Calories	Carbs	Fiber	Protein	Fat
Breakfast					
Lunch					
Dinner					
Snack					
Snack					

Did I reach my carb
allowance with whole foods?   YES   NO

Did I get my minimum
amount of protein today?   YES   NO

Low-carb vegetables

Supplements

Water

Exercise

10,000 Steps

How I Did Today

Weight

DATE _____ DAY   MON.   TUES.   WED.   THURS.   FRI.   SAT.   SUN.

	Calories	Carbs	Fiber	Protein	Fat
Breakfast					
Lunch					
Dinner					
Snack					
Snack					

Did I reach my carb allowance with whole foods? YES NO	Did I get my minimum amount of protein today? YES NO

Low-carb vegetables

Supplements	Water
Exercise	10,000 Steps
How I Did Today	Weight

DATE		DAY	MON.	TUES.	WED.	THURS.	FRI.	SAT.	SUN.

	Calories	Carbs	Fiber	Protein	Fat
Breakfast					
Lunch					
Dinner					
Snack					
Snack					

Did I reach my carb allowance with whole foods? YES NO	Did I get my minimum amount of protein today? YES NO

Low-carb vegetables

Supplements	Water
Exercise	10,000 Steps
How I Did Today	Weight

	Calories	Carbs	Fiber	Protein	Fat
Breakfast					
Lunch					
Dinner					
Snack					
Snack					

DATE _____   **DAY**   MON.   TUES.   WED.   THURS.   FRI.   SAT.   SUN.

Did I reach my carb allowance with whole foods?   YES   NO

Did I get my minimum amount of protein today?   YES   NO

Low-carb vegetables

Supplements

Water

Exercise

10,000 Steps

How I Did Today

Weight

DATE _____ **DAY** MON. TUES. WED. THURS. FRI. SAT. SUN.

	Calories	Carbs	Fiber	Protein	Fat
Breakfast					
Lunch					
Dinner					
Snack					
Snack					

Did I reach my carb allowance with whole foods?　　YES　　NO

Did I get my minimum amount of protein today?　　YES　　NO

Low-carb vegetables

Supplements

Water

Exercise

10,000 Steps

How I Did Today

Weight

	Calories	Carbs	Fiber	Protein	Fat
Breakfast					
Lunch					
Dinner					
Snack					
Snack					

Did I reach my carb allowance with whole foods? YES NO	Did I get my minimum amount of protein today? YES NO

Low-carb vegetables

Supplements	Water
Exercise	10,000 Steps
How I Did Today	Weight

DATE _____ **DAY** MON. TUES. WED. THURS. FRI. SAT. SUN.

	Calories	Carbs	Fiber	Protein	Fat
Breakfast					
Lunch					
Dinner					
Snack					
Snack					

Did I reach my carb allowance with whole foods?   YES   NO

Did I get my minimum amount of protein today?   YES   NO

Low-carb vegetables

Supplements

Water

Exercise

10,000 Steps

How I Did Today

Weight

	Calories	Carbs	Fiber	Protein	Fat
Breakfast					
Lunch					
Dinner					
Snack					
Snack					

Did I reach my carb allowance with whole foods? YES NO	Did I get my minimum amount of protein today? YES NO

Low-carb vegetables

Supplements	Water
Exercise	10,000 Steps
How I Did Today	Weight

DATE _____ **DAY** MON. TUES. WED. THURS. FRI. SAT. SUN.

	Calories	Carbs	Fiber	Protein	Fat
Breakfast					
Lunch					
Dinner					
Snack					
Snack					

Did I reach my carb allowance with whole foods?   YES   NO

Did I get my minimum amount of protein today?   YES   NO

Low-carb vegetables

Supplements

Water

Exercise

10,000 Steps

How I Did Today

Weight

DATE			DAY	MON.	TUES.	WED.	THURS.	FRI.	SAT.	SUN.

	Calories	Carbs	Fiber	Protein	Fat
Breakfast					
Lunch					
Dinner					
Snack					
Snack					

Did I reach my carb allowance with whole foods? YES NO	Did I get my minimum amount of protein today? YES NO

Low-carb vegetables

Supplements	Water
Exercise	10,000 Steps
How I Did Today	Weight

	Calories	Carbs	Fiber	Protein	Fat
Breakfast					
Lunch					
Dinner					
Snack					
Snack					

Did I reach my carb allowance with whole foods?   YES   NO

Did I get my minimum amount of protein today?   YES   NO

Low-carb vegetables

Supplements

Water

Exercise

10,000 Steps

How I Did Today

Weight

DATE _____ / **DAY** MON. TUES. WED. · THURS. FRI. SAT. SUN.
_____

	Calories	Carbs	Fiber	Protein	Fat
Breakfast					
Lunch					
Dinner					
Snack					
Snack					

| Did I reach my carb allowance with whole foods?   YES   NO | Did I get my minimum amount of protein today?   YES   NO |

Low-carb vegetables

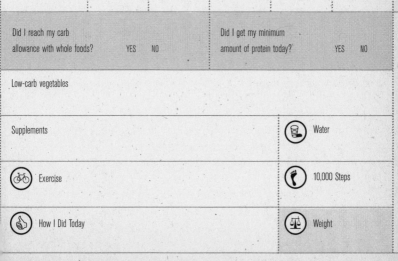

Supplements

Water

Exercise

10,000 Steps

How I Did Today

Weight

DATE _____ **DAY** MON. TUES. WED. THURS. FRI. SAT. SUN.

	Calories	Carbs	Fiber	Protein	Fat
Breakfast					
Lunch					
Dinner					
Snack					
Snack					

Did I reach my carb allowance with whole foods?   YES   NO

Did I get my minimum amount of protein today?   YES   NO

Low-carb vegetables

Supplements

Water

Exercise

10,000 Steps

How I Did Today

Weight

DATE _____ **DAY**   MON.   TUES.   WED.   THURS.   FRI.   SAT.   SUN.

	Calories	Carbs	Fiber	Protein	Fat
Breakfast					
Lunch					
Dinner					
Snack					
Snack					

Did I reach my carb allowance with whole foods?   YES   NO

Did I get my minimum amount of protein today?   YES   NO

Low-carb vegetables

Supplements

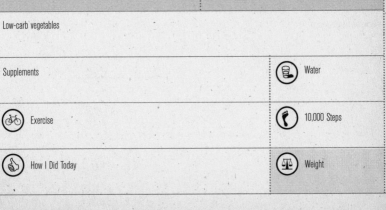

Water

Exercise

10,000 Steps

How I Did Today

Weight

	Calories	Carbs	Fiber	Protein	Fat
Breakfast					
Lunch					
Dinner					
Snack					
Snack					

Did I reach my carb allowance with whole foods? YES NO	Did I get my minimum amount of protein today? YES NO

Low-carb vegetables

Supplements	Water
Exercise	10,000 Steps
How I Did Today	Weight

DATE _____ **DAY**   MON.   TUES.   WED.   THURS.   FRI.   SAT.   SUN.

	Calories	Carbs	Fiber	Protein	Fat
Breakfast					
Lunch					
Dinner					
Snack					
Snack					

Did I reach my carb allowance with whole foods?   YES   NO

Did I get my minimum amount of protein today?   YES   NO

Low-carb vegetables

Supplements

Water

Exercise

10,000 Steps

How I Did Today

Weight

	Calories	Carbs	Fiber	Protein	Fat
Breakfast					
Lunch					
Dinner					
Snack					
Snack					

Did I reach my carb allowance with whole foods? YES NO	Did I get my minimum amount of protein today? YES NO

Low-carb vegetables

Supplements	Water
Exercise	10,000 Steps
How I Did Today	Weight

DATE			**DAY**	MON. TUES. WED. THURS. FRI. SAT. SUN.	

	Calories	Carbs	Fiber	Protein	Fat
Breakfast					
Lunch					
Dinner					
Snack					
Snack					

Did I reach my carb allowance with whole foods?   YES   NO

Did I get my minimum amount of protein today?   YES   NO

Low-carb vegetables

Supplements

Water

Exercise

10,000 Steps

How I Did Today

Weight

DATE _____   **DAY**   MON.   TUES.   WED.   THURS.   FRI.   SAT.   SUN.

	Calories	Carbs	Fiber	Protein	Fat
Breakfast					
Lunch					
Dinner					
Snack					
Snack					

Did I reach my carb allowance with whole foods?   YES   NO

Did I get my minimum amount of protein today?   YES   NO

Low-carb vegetables

Supplements

Water

Exercise

10,000 Steps

How I Did Today

Weight

	Calories	Carbs	Fiber	Protein	Fat
Breakfast					
Lunch					
Dinner					
Snack					
Snack					

Did I reach my carb allowance with whole foods?   YES   NO

Did I get my minimum amount of protein today?   YES   NO

Low-carb vegetables

Supplements

Water

Exercise

10,000 Steps

How I Did Today

Weight

	Calories	Carbs	Fiber	Protein	Fat
Breakfast					
Lunch					
Dinner					
Snack					
Snack					

Did I reach my carb allowance with whole foods?   YES   NO

Did I get my minimum amount of protein today?   YES   NO

Low-carb vegetables

Supplements   Water

Exercise   10,000 Steps

How I Did Today   Weight

DATE _____ **DAY** MON. TUES. WED. THURS. FRI. SAT. SUN.

	Calories	Carbs	Fiber	Protein	Fat
Breakfast					
Lunch					
Dinner					
Snack					
Snack					

Did I reach my carb
allowance with whole foods?   YES   NO

Did I get my minimum
amount of protein today?   YES   NO

Low-carb vegetables

Supplements

Water

Exercise

10,000 Steps

How I Did Today

Weight

	Calories	Carbs	Fiber	Protein	Fat
Breakfast					
Lunch					
Dinner					
Snack					
Snack					

Did I reach my carb allowance with whole foods? YES NO	Did I get my minimum amount of protein today? YES NO

Low-carb vegetables

Supplements	Water
Exercise	10,000 Steps
How I Did Today	Weight

	Calories	Carbs	Fiber	Protein	Fat
Breakfast					
Lunch					
Dinner					
Snack					
Snack					

Did I reach my carb allowance with whole foods?   YES   NO

Did I get my minimum amount of protein today?   YES   NO

Low-carb vegetables

Supplements   Water

Exercise   10,000 Steps

How I Did Today   Weight

	Calories	Carbs	Fiber	Protein	Fat
DATE					

DATE DAY MON. TUES. WED. THURS. FRI. SAT. SUN.

	Calories	Carbs	Fiber	Protein	Fat
Breakfast					
Lunch					
Dinner					
Snack					
Snack					

Did I reach my carb allowance with whole foods? YES NO	Did I get my minimum amount of protein today? YES NO

Low-carb vegetables

Supplements	Water
Exercise	10,000 Steps
How I Did Today	Weight

DATE   **DAY**   MON.   TUES.   WED.   THURS.   FRI.   SAT.   SUN.

	Calories	Carbs	Fiber	Protein	Fat
Breakfast					
Lunch					
Dinner					
Snack					
Snack					

Did I reach my carb
allowance with whole foods?   YES   NO

Did I get my minimum
amount of protein today?   YES   NO

Low-carb vegetables

Supplements

Water

Exercise

10,000 Steps

How I Did Today

Weight

	Calories	Carbs	Fiber	Protein	Fat
DATE		**DAY** MON. TUES. WED. THURS. FRI. SAT. SUN.			

	Calories	Carbs	Fiber	Protein	Fat
Breakfast					
Lunch					
Dinner					
Snack					
Snack					

Did I reach my carb allowance with whole foods?   YES   NO

Did I get my minimum amount of protein today?   YES   NO

Low-carb vegetables

Supplements

Water

Exercise

10,000 Steps

How I Did Today

Weight

DATE		DAY	MON.	TUES.	WED.	THURS.	FRI.	SAT.	SUN.

	Calories	Carbs	Fiber	Protein	Fat
Breakfast					
Lunch					
Dinner					
Snack					
Snack					

Did I reach my carb allowance with whole foods? YES NO	Did I get my minimum amount of protein today? YES NO

Low-carb vegetables

Supplements	Water
Exercise	10,000 Steps
How I Did Today	Weight

DATE _____ **DAY**   MON.   TUES.   WED.   THURS.   FRI.   SAT.   SUN.

	Calories	Carbs	Fiber	Protein	Fat
Breakfast					
Lunch					
Dinner					
Snack					
Snack					

Did I reach my carb allowance with whole foods? YES NO	Did I get my minimum amount of protein today? YES NO

Low-carb vegetables

Supplements	Water
Exercise	10,000 Steps
How I Did Today	Weight

DATE				**DAY**	MON.	TUES.	WED.	THURS.	FRI.	SAT.	SUN.

	Calories	Carbs	Fiber	Protein	Fat
Breakfast					
Lunch					
Dinner					
Snack					
Snack					

Did I reach my carb
allowance with whole foods?   YES   NO

Did I get my minimum
amount of protein today?   YES   NO

Low-carb vegetables

Supplements

 Water

 Exercise

 10,000 Steps

 How I Did Today

 Weight

DATE _____ **DAY** MON. TUES. WED. THURS. FRI. SAT. SUN.

	Calories	Carbs	Fiber	Protein	Fat
Breakfast					
Lunch					
Dinner					
Snack					
Snack					

Did I reach my carb allowance with whole foods? YES NO	Did I get my minimum amount of protein today? YES NO

Low-carb vegetables

Supplements	Water
Exercise	10,000 Steps
How I Did Today	Weight

	Calories	Carbs	Fiber	Protein	Fat
Breakfast					
Lunch					
Dinner					
Snack					
Snack					

Did I reach my carb allowance with whole foods? YES NO	Did I get my minimum amount of protein today? YES NO

Low-carb vegetables

Supplements	Water
Exercise	10,000 Steps
How I Did Today	Weight

DATE _____ **DAY**   MON.   TUES.   WED.   THURS.   FRI.   SAT.   SUN.

	Calories	Carbs	Fiber	Protein	Fat
Breakfast					
Lunch					
Dinner					
Snack					
Snack					

Did I reach my carb allowance with whole foods?   YES   NO

Did I get my minimum amount of protein today?   YES   NO

Low-carb vegetables

Supplements

Water

Exercise

10,000 Steps

How I Did Today

Weight

DATE _____   **DAY**   MON.   TUES.   WED.   THURS.   FRI.   SAT.   SUN.

	Calories	Carbs	Fiber	Protein	Fat
Breakfast					
Lunch					
Dinner					
Snack					
Snack					

Did I reach my carb
allowance with whole foods?   YES   NO

Did I get my minimum
amount of protein today?   YES   NO

Low-carb vegetables

Supplements

Water

Exercise

10,000 Steps

How I Did Today

Weight

	Calories	Carbs	Fiber	Protein	Fat
DATE			**DAY** MON. TUES. WED. THURS. FRI. SAT. SUN.		

	Calories	Carbs	Fiber	Protein	Fat
Breakfast					
Lunch					
Dinner					
Snack					
Snack					

Did I reach my carb allowance with whole foods?   YES   NO

Did I get my minimum amount of protein today?   YES   NO

Low-carb vegetables.

Supplements

Water

Exercise

10,000 Steps

How I Did Today

Weight

	Calories	Carbs	Fiber	Protein	Fat
Breakfast					
Lunch					
Dinner					
Snack					
Snack					

Did I reach my carb
allowance with whole foods?   YES   NO

Did I get my minimum
amount of protein today?   YES   NO

Low-carb vegetables

Supplements

Water

Exercise

10,000 Steps

How I Did Today

Weight

	Calories	Carbs	Fiber	Protein	Fat
Breakfast					
Lunch					
Dinner					
Snack					
Snack					

Did I reach my carb allowance with whole foods? YES NO	Did I get my minimum amount of protein today? YES NO

Low-carb vegetables

Supplements	Water
Exercise	10,000 Steps
How I Did Today	Weight

DATE _____   **DAY**   MON.   TUES.   WED.   THURS.   FRI.   SAT.   SUN.

	Calories	Carbs	Fiber	Protein	Fat
Breakfast					
Lunch					
Dinner					
Snack					
Snack					

Did I reach my carb
allowance with whole foods?   YES   NO

Did I get my minimum
amount of protein today?   YES   NO

Low-carb vegetables

Supplements

Water

Exercise

10,000 Steps

How I Did Today

Weight

DATE			DAY	MON.	TUES.	WED.	THURS.	FRI.	SAT.	SUN.

	Calories	Carbs	Fiber	Protein	Fat
Breakfast					
Lunch					
Dinner					
Snack					
Snack					

Did I reach my carb allowance with whole foods? YES NO	Did I get my minimum amount of protein today? YES NO

Low-carb vegetables

Supplements	Water
Exercise	10,000 Steps
How I Did Today	Weight

DATE _____ **DAY**   MON.   TUES.   WED.   THURS.   FRI.   SAT.   SUN.

	Calories	Carbs	Fiber	Protein	Fat
Breakfast					
Lunch					
Dinner					
Snack					
Snack					

Did I reach my carb allowance with whole foods? YES NO	Did I get my minimum amount of protein today? YES NO

Low-carb vegetables

Supplements	Water
Exercise	10,000 Steps
How I Did Today	Weight

DATE   **DAY**   MON.   TUES.   WED.   THURS.   FRI.   SAT.   SUN.

	Calories	Carbs	Fiber	Protein	Fat
Breakfast					
Lunch					
Dinner					
Snack					
Snack					

Did I reach my carb allowance with whole foods? YES NO	Did I get my minimum amount of protein today? YES NO	

Low-carb vegetables

Supplements	Water
Exercise	10,000 Steps
How I Did Today	Weight

	Calories	Carbs	Fiber	Protein	Fat
Breakfast					
Lunch					
Dinner					
Snack					
Snack					

Did I reach my carb allowance with whole foods?　　YES　NO

Did I get my minimum amount of protein today?　　YES　NO

Low-carb vegetables

Supplements

Water

Exercise

10,000 Steps

How I Did Today

Weight

	Calories	Carbs	Fiber	Protein	Fat
Breakfast					
Lunch					
Dinner					
Snack					
Snack					

Did I reach my carb allowance with whole foods? YES NO	Did I get my minimum amount of protein today? YES NO

Low-carb vegetables

Supplements	Water
Exercise	10,000 Steps
How I Did Today	Weight

DATE _____ **DAY**   MON.   TUES.   WED.   THURS.   FRI.   SAT.   SUN.

	Calories	Carbs	Fiber	Protein	Fat
Breakfast					
Lunch					
Dinner					
Snack					
Snack					

Did I reach my carb
allowance with whole foods?   YES   NO

Did I get my minimum
amount of protein today?   YES   NO

Low-carb vegetables

Supplements

Water

Exercise

10,000 Steps

How I Did Today

Weight

DATE _____   **DAY**   MON.   TUES.   WED.   THURS.   FRI.   SAT.   SUN.

	Calories	Carbs	Fiber	Protein	Fat
Breakfast					
Lunch					
Dinner					
Snack					
Snack					

Did I reach my carb allowance with whole foods? YES NO	Did I get my minimum amount of protein today? YES NO

Low-carb vegetables

Supplements	Water
Exercise	10,000 Steps
How I Did Today	Weight

DATE .... **DAY** MON.   TUES.   WED.   THURS.   FRI.   SAT.   SUN.

	Calories	Carbs	Fiber	Protein	Fat
Breakfast					
Lunch					
Dinner					
Snack					
Snack					

Did I reach my carb allowance with whole foods? YES NO	Did I get my minimum amount of protein today? YES NO

Low-carb vegetables

Supplements	Water
Exercise	10,000 Steps
How I Did Today	Weight

DATE _____ **DAY** MON. TUES. WED. THURS. FRI. SAT. SUN.

	Calories	Carbs	Fiber	Protein	Fat
Breakfast					
Lunch					
Dinner					
Snack					
Snack					

Did I reach my carb allowance with whole foods? YES NO	Did I get my minimum amount of protein today? YES NO

Low-carb vegetables

Supplements	Water
Exercise	10,000 Steps
How I Did Today	Weight

DATE		**DAY**	MON.	TUES.	WED.	THURS.	FRI.	SAT.	SUN.

	Calories	Carbs	Fiber	Protein	Fat
Breakfast					
Lunch					
Dinner					
Snack					
Snack					

Did I reach my carb allowance with whole foods?	YES	NO	Did I get my minimum amount of protein today?	YES	NO

Low-carb vegetables

Supplements	Water
Exercise	10,000 Steps
How I Did Today	Weight

DATE _____ **DAY**   MON.   TUES.   WED.   THURS.   FRI.   SAT.   SUN.

	Calories	Carbs	Fiber	Protein	Fat
Breakfast					
Lunch					
Dinner					
Snack					
Snack					

Did I reach my carb allowance with whole foods? YES NO	Did I get my minimum amount of protein today? YES NO

Low-carb vegetables _____

Supplements	Water
Exercise	10,000 Steps
How I Did Today	Weight

	Calories	Carbs	Fiber	Protein	Fat
Breakfast					
Lunch					
Dinner					
Snack					
Snack					

Did I reach my carb allowance with whole foods? YES NO	Did I get my minimum amount of protein today? YES NO	

Low-carb vegetables

Supplements	Water
Exercise	10,000 Steps
How I Did Today	Weight

DATE		**DAY**	MON.	TUES.	WED.	THURS.	FRI.	SAT.	SUN.

	Calories	Carbs	Fiber	Protein	Fat
Breakfast					
Lunch					
Dinner					
Snack					
Snack					

Did I reach my carb allowance with whole foods? YES NO	Did I get my minimum amount of protein today? YES NO

Low-carb vegetables

Supplements	Water
Exercise	10,000 Steps
How I Did Today	Weight

DATE		**DAY**	MON.	TUES.	WED.	THURS.	FRI.	SAT.	SUN.

	Calories	Carbs	Fiber	Protein	Fat
Breakfast					
Lunch					
Dinner					
Snack					
Snack					

Did I reach my carb allowance with whole foods? YES NO	Did I get my minimum amount of protein today? YES NO

Low-carb vegetables

Supplements	Water
Exercise	10,000 Steps
How I Did Today	Weight

DATE _____ **DAY** MON. TUES. WED. THURS. FRI. SAT. SUN.

	Calories	Carbs	Fiber	Protein	Fat
Breakfast					
Lunch					
Dinner					
Snack					
Snack					

Did I reach my carb allowance with whole foods? YES NO	Did I get my minimum amount of protein today? YES NO

Low-carb vegetables

Supplements	Water
Exercise	10,000 Steps
How I Did Today	Weight

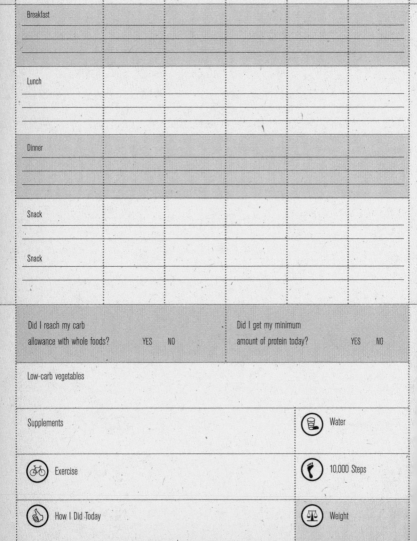

DATE _____ **DAY** MON. TUES. WED. THURS. FRI. SAT. SUN.

	Calories	Carbs	Fiber	Protein	Fat
Breakfast					
Lunch					
Dinner					
Snack					
Snack					

Did I reach my carb allowance with whole foods? YES NO	Did I get my minimum amount of protein today? YES NO

Low-carb vegetables

Supplements	Water
Exercise	10,000 Steps
How I Did Today	Weight

DATE				DAY	MON.	TUES.	WED.	THURS.	FRI.	SAT.	SUN.

	Calories	Carbs	Fiber	Protein	Fat
Breakfast					
Lunch					
Dinner					
Snack					
Snack					

Did I reach my carb allowance with whole foods?　YES　NO

Did I get my minimum amount of protein today?　YES　NO

Low-carb vegetables

Supplements

Water

Exercise

10,000 Steps

How I Did Today

Weight

	Calories	Carbs	Fiber	Protein	Fat
DATE		**DAY** MON. TUES. WED. THURS. FRI. SAT. SUN.			

	Calories	Carbs	Fiber	Protein	Fat
Breakfast					
Lunch					
Dinner					
Snack					
Snack					

Did I reach my carb allowance with whole foods?	YES	NO	Did I get my minimum amount of protein today?	YES	NO

Low-carb vegetables

Supplements

Water

Exercise

10,000 Steps

How I Did Today

Weight

	Calories	Carbs	Fiber	Protein	Fat
Breakfast					
Lunch					
Dinner					
Snack					
Snack					

Did I reach my carb allowance with whole foods? YES NO	Did I get my minimum amount of protein today? YES NO

Low-carb vegetables

Supplements	Water
Exercise	10,000 Steps
How I Did Today	Weight

	Calories	Carbs	Fiber	Protein	Fat
Breakfast					
Lunch					
Dinner					
Snack					
Snack					

Did I reach my carb allowance with whole foods? YES NO	Did I get my minimum amount of protein today? YES NO

Low-carb vegetables

Supplements	Water
Exercise	10,000 Steps
How I Did Today	Weight

DATE		**DAY**	MON.	TUES.	WED.	THURS.	FRI.	SAT.	SUN.

	Calories	Carbs	Fiber	Protein	Fat
Breakfast					
Lunch					
Dinner					
Snack					
Snack					

Did I reach my carb allowance with whole foods? YES NO	Did I get my minimum amount of protein today? YES NO

Low-carb vegetables

Supplements	Water
Exercise	10,000 Steps
How I Did Today	Weight

| DATE | | | DAY | MON. | TUES. | WED. | THURS. | FRI. | SAT. | SUN. |

	Calories	Carbs	Fiber	Protein	Fat
Breakfast					
Lunch					
Dinner					
Snack					
Snack					

Did I reach my carb allowance with whole foods?   YES   NO

Did I get my minimum amount of protein today?   YES   NO

Low-carb vegetables

Supplements

Water

Exercise

10,000 Steps

How I Did Today

Weight

	Calories	Carbs	Fiber	Protein	Fat
Breakfast					
Lunch					
Dinner					
Snack					
Snack					

DATE _____ **DAY** MON. TUES. WED. THURS. FRI. SAT. SUN.

Did I reach my carb allowance with whole foods?   YES   NO

Did I get my minimum amount of protein today?   YES   NO

Low-carb vegetables

Supplements

Water

Exercise

10,000 Steps

How I Did Today

Weight

DATE _____ **DAY** MON. TUES. WED. THURS. FRI. SAT. SUN.

	Calories	Carbs	Fiber	Protein	Fat
Breakfast					
Lunch					
Dinner					
Snack					
Snack					

Did I reach my carb
allowance with whole foods?   YES   NO

Did I get my minimum
amount of protein today?   YES   NO

Low-carb vegetables

Supplements

 Water

 Exercise

 10,000 Steps

 How I Did Today

 Weight

	Calories	Carbs	Fiber	Protein	Fat
Breakfast					
Lunch					
Dinner					
Snack					
Snack					

Did I reach my carb
allowance with whole foods?   YES   NO

Did I get my minimum
amount of protein today?   YES   NO

Low-carb vegetables

Supplements

Water

Exercise

10,000 Steps

How I Did Today

Weight

DATE _____ **DAY**   MON.   TUES.   WED.   THURS.   FRI.   SAT.   SUN.

	Calories	Carbs	Fiber	Protein	Fat
Breakfast					
Lunch					
Dinner					
Snack					
Snack					

Did I reach my carb allowance with whole foods? YES NO	Did I get my minimum amount of protein today? YES NO

Low-carb vegetables

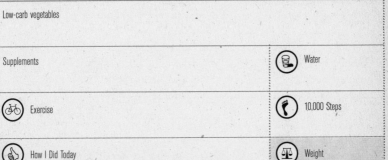

Supplements	Water
Exercise	10,000 Steps
How I Did Today	Weight

	Calories	Carbs	Fiber	Protein	Fat
Breakfast					
Lunch					
Dinner					
Snack					
Snack					

Did I reach my carb allowance with whole foods? YES NO	Did I get my minimum amount of protein today? YES NO

Low-carb vegetables

Supplements	Water
Exercise	10,000 Steps
How I Did Today	Weight

	Calories	Carbs	Fiber	Protein	Fat
Breakfast					
Lunch					
Dinner					
Snack					
Snack					

Did I reach my carb allowance with whole foods?   YES   NO

Did I get my minimum amount of protein today?   -YES   NO

Low-carb vegetables

Supplements

Water

Exercise

10,000 Steps

How I Did Today

Weight

	Calories	Carbs	Fiber	Protein	Fat
Breakfast					
Lunch					
Dinner					
Snack					
Snack					

Did I reach my carb allowance with whole foods? YES NO	Did I get my minimum amount of protein today? YES NO

Low-carb vegetables

Supplements	Water
Exercise	10,000 Steps
How I Did Today	Weight

DATE _____ **DAY** MON. TUES. WED. THURS. FRI. SAT. SUN.

	Calories	Carbs	Fiber	Protein	Fat
Breakfast					
Lunch					
Dinner					
Snack					
Snack					

Did I reach my carb allowance with whole foods? YES NO	Did I get my minimum amount of protein today? YES NO

Low-carb vegetables

Supplements	Water
Exercise	10,000 Steps
How I Did Today	Weight

	Calories	Carbs	Fiber	Protein	Fat
Breakfast					
Lunch					
Dinner					
Snack					
Snack					

Did I reach my carb allowance with whole foods? YES NO	Did I get my minimum amount of protein today? YES NO

Low-carb vegetables

Supplements	Water
Exercise	10,000 Steps
How I Did Today	Weight

	Calories	Carbs	Fiber	Protein	Fat
Breakfast					
Lunch					
Dinner					
Snack					
Snack					

Did I reach my carb allowance with whole foods?   YES   NO

Did I get my minimum amount of protein today?   YES   NO

Low-carb vegetables

Supplements

Water

Exercise

10,000 Steps

How I Did Today

Weight

DATE _____ **DAY** MON.   TUES.   WED.   THURS.   FRI.   SAT.   SUN.

	Calories	Carbs	Fiber	Protein	Fat
Breakfast					
Lunch					
Dinner					
Snack					
Snack					

Did I reach my carb allowance with whole foods? YES NO	Did I get my minimum amount of protein today? YES NO

Low-carb vegetables

Supplements	Water
Exercise	10,000 Steps
How I Did Today	Weight

	Calories	Carbs	Fiber	Protein	Fat
Breakfast					
Lunch					
Dinner					
Snack					
Snack					

Did I reach my carb allowance with whole foods? YES NO	Did I get my minimum amount of protein today? YES NO

Low-carb vegetables

Supplements	Water
Exercise	10,000 Steps
How I Did Today	Weight

	Calories	Carbs	Fiber	Protein	Fat
DATE _____			**DAY** MON. TUES. WED. THURS. FRI. SAT. SUN.		

	Calories	Carbs	Fiber	Protein	Fat
Breakfast					
Lunch					
Dinner					
Snack					
Snack					

Did I reach my carb allowance with whole foods? YES NO	Did I get my minimum amount of protein today? YES NO

Low-carb vegetables

Supplements	Water
Exercise	10,000 Steps
How I Did Today	Weight

DATE _____ **DAY** MON. TUES. WED. THURS. FRI. SAT. SUN.

	Calories	Carbs	Fiber	Protein	Fat
Breakfast					
Lunch					
Dinner					
Snack					
Snack					

Did I reach my carb allowance with whole foods?   YES   NO

Did I get my minimum amount of protein today?   YES   NO

Low-carb vegetables

Supplements

Water

Exercise

10,000 Steps

How I Did Today

Weight

DATE _____ **DAY**   MON.   TUES.   WED.   THURS.   FRI.   SAT.   SUN.

	Calories	Carbs	Fiber	Protein	Fat
Breakfast					
Lunch					
Dinner					
Snack					
Snack					

Did I reach my carb allowance with whole foods? YES NO	Did I get my minimum amount of protein today? YES NO

Low-carb vegetables

Supplements	Water
Exercise	10,000 Steps
How I Did Today	Weight

	Calories	Carbs	Fiber	Protein	Fat
Breakfast					
Lunch					
Dinner					
Snack					
Snack					

Did I reach my carb allowance with whole foods?   YES   NO

Did I get my minimum amount of protein today?   YES   NO

Low-carb vegetables

Supplements

Water

Exercise

10,000 Steps

How I Did Today

Weight

	Calories	Carbs	Fiber	Protein	Fat
Breakfast					
Lunch					
Dinner					
Snack					
Snack					

Did I reach my carb allowance with whole foods?   YES   NO

Did I get my minimum amount of protein today?   YES   NO

Low-carb vegetables

Supplements

Water

Exercise

10,000 Steps

How I Did Today

Weight

	Calories	Carbs	Fiber	Protein	Fat
DATE _____ **DAY** MON. TUES. WED. THURS. FRI. SAT. SUN.					

	Calories	Carbs	Fiber	Protein	Fat
Breakfast					
Lunch					
Dinner					
Snack					
Snack					

Did I reach my carb allowance with whole foods?   YES   NO

Did I get my minimum amount of protein today?   YES   NO

Low-carb vegetables

Supplements

Water

Exercise

10,000 Steps

How I Did Today

Weight

DATE		DAY	MON.	TUES.	WED.	THURS.	FRI.	SAT.	SUN.

	Calories	Carbs	Fiber	Protein	Fat	
Breakfast						
Lunch						
Dinner						
Snack						
Snack						

Did I reach my carb allowance with whole foods?	YES	NO	Did I get my minimum amount of protein today?	YES	NO

Low-carb vegetables

Supplements		Water
Exercise		10,000 Steps
How I Did Today		Weight

DATE _____   **DAY**   MON.   TUES.   WED.   THURS.   FRI.   SAT.   SUN.

	Calories	Carbs	Fiber	Protein	Fat
Breakfast					
Lunch					
Dinner					
Snack					
Snack					

Did I reach my carb allowance with whole foods? YES NO	Did I get my minimum amount of protein today? YES NO

Low-carb vegetables

Supplements   Water

Exercise   10,000 Steps

How I Did Today   Weight

	Calories	Carbs	Fiber	Protein	Fat
Breakfast					
Lunch					
Dinner					
Snack					
Snack					

| Did I reach my carb allowance with whole foods?   YES   NO | Did I get my minimum amount of protein today?   YES   NO |

Low-carb vegetables

Supplements	Water
Exercise	10,000 Steps
How I Did Today	Weight

	Calories	Carbs	Fiber	Protein	Fat
Breakfast					
Lunch					
Dinner					
Snack					
Snack					

DATE _____ **DAY**   MON.   TUES.   WED.   THURS.   FRI.   SAT.   SUN.

Did I reach my carb allowance with whole foods?   YES   NO

Did I get my minimum amount of protein today?   YES   NO

Low-carb vegetables

Supplements

Water

Exercise

10,000 Steps

How I Did Today

Weight

DATE   **DAY**   MON.   TUES.   WED.   THURS.   FRI.   SAT.   SUN.

	Calories	Carbs	Fiber	Protein	Fat
Breakfast					
Lunch					
Dinner					
Snack					
Snack					

Did I reach my carb allowance with whole foods? YES NO	Did I get my minimum amount of protein today? YES NO

Low-carb vegetables

Supplements	Water
Exercise	10,000 Steps
How I Did Today	Weight

DAY   MON.   TUES.   WED.   THURS.   FRI.   SAT.   SUN.

	Calories	Carbs	Fiber	Protein	Fat
Breakfast					
Lunch					
Dinner					
Snack					
Snack					

Did I reach my carb allowance with whole foods? YES NO	Did I get my minimum amount of protein today? YES NO

Low-carb vegetables

Supplements	Water
Exercise	10,000 Steps
How I Did Today	Weight

| DATE | | **DAY** | MON. | TUES. | WED. | THURS. | FRI. | SAT. | SUN. |

	Calories	Carbs	Fiber	Protein	Fat
Breakfast					
Lunch					
Dinner					
Snack					
Snack					

Did I reach my carb allowance with whole foods? YES NO	Did I get my minimum amount of protein today? YES NO

Low-carb vegetables

Supplements	Water
Exercise	10,000 Steps
How I Did Today	Weight

DATE _____   **DAY**   MON.   TUES.   WED.   THURS.   FRI.   SAT.   SUN.

	Calories	Carbs	Fiber	Protein	Fat
Breakfast					
Lunch					
Dinner					
Snack					
Snack					

Did I reach my carb allowance with whole foods? YES NO	Did I get my minimum amount of protein today? YES NO

Low-carb vegetables

Supplements	Water
Exercise	10,000 Steps
How I Did Today	Weight

	Calories	Carbs	Fiber	Protein	Fat
Breakfast					
Lunch					
Dinner					
Snack					
Snack					

Did I reach my carb allowance with whole foods? YES NO	Did I get my minimum amount of protein today? YES NO

Low-carb vegetables

Supplements	Water
Exercise	10,000 Steps
How I Did Today	Weight

DATE   **DAY**   MON.   TUES.   WED.   THURS.   FRI.   SAT.   SUN.

	Calories	Carbs	Fiber	Protein	Fat
Breakfast					
Lunch					
Dinner					
Snack					
Snack					

Did I reach my carb allowance with whole foods? YES NO	Did I get my minimum amount of protein today? YES NO

Low-carb vegetables

Supplements	Water
Exercise	10,000 Steps
How I Did Today	Weight

DATE _____   **DAY**   MON.   TUES.   WED.   THURS.   FRI.   SAT.   SUN.

	Calories	Carbs	Fiber	Protein	Fat
Breakfast					
Lunch					
Dinner					
Snack					
Snack					

Did I reach my carb
allowance with whole foods?   YES   NO

Did I get my minimum
amount of protein today?   YES   NO

Low-carb vegetables

Supplements   Water

Exercise   10,000 Steps

How I Did Today   Weight

DATE _____ **DAY**   MON.   TUES.   WED.   THURS.   FRI.   SAT.   SUN.

	Calories	Carbs	Fiber	Protein	Fat
Breakfast					
Lunch					
Dinner					
Snack					
Snack					

Did I reach my carb allowance with whole foods?   YES   NO

Did I get my minimum amount of protein today?   YES   NO

Low-carb vegetables

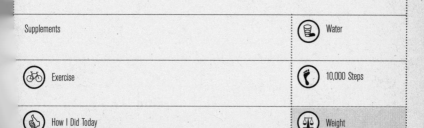

Supplements

Water

Exercise

10,000 Steps

How I Did Today

Weight

	Calories	Carbs	Fiber	Protein	Fat	
Breakfast						
Lunch						
Dinner						
Snack						
Snack						

DATE _____ **DAY**   MON.   TUES.   WED.   THURS.   FRI.   SAT.   SUN.

Did I reach my carb allowance with whole foods?   YES   NO

Did I get my minimum amount of protein today?   YES   NO

Low-carb vegetables

Supplements

Water

Exercise

10,000 Steps

How I Did Today

Weight

	Calories	Carbs	Fiber	Protein	Fat
Breakfast					
Lunch					
Dinner					
Snack					
Snack					

Did I reach my carb allowance with whole foods? YES NO	Did I get my minimum amount of protein today? YES NO

Low-carb vegetables

Supplements	Water
Exercise	10,000 Steps
How I Did Today	Weight

DATE		**DAY**	MON.	TUES.	WED.	THURS.	FRI.	SAT.	SUN.

	Calories	Carbs	Fiber	Protein	Fat
Breakfast					
Lunch					
Dinner					
Snack					
Snack					

Did I reach my carb allowance with whole foods? YES NO	Did I get my minimum amount of protein today? YES NO

Low-carb vegetables

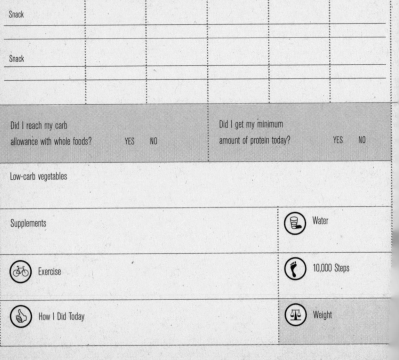

Supplements

Water

Exercise

10,000 Steps

How I Did Today

Weight

	Calories	Carbs	Fiber	Protein.	Fat
Breakfast					
Lunch					
Dinner					
Snack					
Snack					

Did I reach my carb allowance with whole foods? YES NO	Did I get my minimum amount of protein today? YES NO

Low-carb vegetables

Supplements	Water
Exercise	10,000 Steps
How I Did Today	Weight

Nutritional Information for Popular Foods

	SERVING SIZE	CALORIES	TOTAL CARBS (g)	FIBER (g)	PROTEIN (g)	FAT (g)
BEVERAGES						
Apple juice	8 fl oz	115	29	Tr	Tr	Tr
Beer, regular	12 fl oz	150	13	1	1	0
Light beer	12 fl oz	100	6	0	1	0
Malt beer	12 fl oz	160	10	Tr	1	0
Capri Sun juice drink	8 fl oz	122	31	Tr	Tr	Tr
Carrot juice	8 fl oz	95	22	2	2	Tr
Club soda	12 fl oz	0	0	0	0	0
Coffee, regular or decaf	6 fl oz	4	1	0	Tr	0
Cappuccino	6 fl oz	65	6	0	3	3
Espresso	2 fl oz	5	1	0	Tr	Tr
Cranberry juice cocktail	8 fl oz	145	36	Tr	0	Tr
Creamers						
Half and half (cream and milk)	1 tbsp	20	1	0	1	2
Liquid creamer *Coffee-Mate*	1 tbsp	20	2	0	Tr	1
Powdered creamer *Coffee-Mate*	1 tsp	10	2	0	Tr	Tr
Crystal Light, all flavors	8 fl oz	5	0	0	0	0
Daiquiri, strawberry	4 fl oz	225	8	Tr	Tr	Tr
Gin 80 proof	1.5 fl oz	95	0	0	0	0
Grapefruit juice, fresh squeezed, unsweetened	8 fl oz	95	22	Tr	1	Tr
Hot chocolate, sugar free	6 fl oz	35	5	Tr	3	0
Lemonade, sweetened	8 fl oz	100	25	Tr	0	0
Margarita	5 fl oz	150	10	Tr	0	0
Martini	2.5 fl oz	155	0	0	0	0

	SERVING SIZE	CALORIES	TOTAL CARBS (g)	FIBER (g)	PROTEIN (g)	FAT (g)
Milk						
Whole milk, 3.3% fat	8 fl oz	150	11	0	8	8
Reduced fat milk, 2% fat	8 fl oz	120	12	0	8	5
Lowfat milk, 1% fat	8 fl oz	102	12	0	8	3
Nonfat milk, (skim milk)	8 fl oz	85	12	0	8	Tr
Whole chocolate milk	8 fl oz	210	26	2	8	8
Reduced fat chocolate milk, 2%	8 fl oz	180	26	1	8	5
Lowfat chocolate milk, 1%	8 fl oz	160	26	1	8	3
Soy milk	1 cup	81	4	3	7	5
Orange juice						
Fresh squeezed, unsweetened	8 fl oz	112	26	1	2	Tr
Canned or bottled, unsweetened	8 fl oz	110	25	1	2	Tr
Frozen concentrate	8 fl oz	112	26	1	2	Tr
Pina colada	4.5 fl oz	260	40	1	1	3
Rum 80 proof	1.5 fl oz	95	0	0	0	0
Scotch 80 proof	1.5 fl oz	95	0	0	0	0
Tequila	1.5 fl oz	100	0	0	0	0
Tomato juice	8 fl oz	41	10	1	2	Tr
V8 Vegetable Juice, 1 large can	11.5 fl oz	70	15	2	2	Tr
Vodka 80 proof	1.5 fl oz	95	0	0	0	0
Water	8 fl oz	0	0	0	0	0
Whiskey 80 proof	1.5 fl oz	95	0	0	0	0
Wine						
Dessert wine, dry	4 fl oz	150	5	0	Tr	0
Dessert wine, sweet	4 fl oz	180	14	0	Tr	0
Red wine (table wine)	4 fl oz	85	2	0	Tr	0

	SERVING SIZE	CALORIES	TOTAL CARBS (g)	FIBER (g)	PROTEIN (g)	FAT (g)
Rosé wine	4 fl oz	85	1	0	Tr	0
White wine (table wine)	4 fl oz	80	1	0	Tr	0
White Zinfandel	4 fl oz	85	1	0	Tr	0
Wine cooler	5.5 fl oz	100	11	0	Tr	0
Wine spritzer	5.5 fl oz	60	1	0	Tr	0

FOODS

	SERVING SIZE	CALORIES	TOTAL CARBS (g)	FIBER (g)	PROTEIN (g)	FAT (g)
Apple, fresh unpeeled	1	80	21	4	Tr	Tr
Apricot fresh, medium size, 1.3 oz	1	17	4	1	Tr	Tr
Apricot dried, halves	10 halves	85	22	3	1	Tr
Arugula, raw	1/2 cup	3	Tr	Tr	Tr	0
Asparagus fresh, medium size spears	4 spears	14	3	1	2	Tr
Chopped pieces	1 cup	43	8	3	5	1
Aspartame Sweetener	1 pkt	0	Tr	0	0	0
Avocado California, 1/5 of whole	1 oz	50	2	1	1	5
Banana, fresh, 7" long	1	110	28	3	1	1
Beans						
Black beans	1/2 cup	115	21	8	7	1
Baked beans, plain or vegetarian	1/2 cup	118	26	6	6	1
Great Northern beans	1/2 cup	105	19	6	7	1
Green beans	1/2 cup	22	5	3	1	Tr
Kidney, red beans	1/2 cup	112	20	7	7	1
Lima, large beans	1/2 cup	100	17	8	7	1
Lima, baby lima beans	1/2 cup	95	17	10	6	1
Pinto beans	1/2 cup	117	22	7	7	1
Soybeans	1/2 cup	135	10	5	12	6

	SERVING SIZE	CALORIES	TOTAL CARBS (g)	FIBER (g)	PROTEIN (g)	FAT (g)
Wax beans	1/2 cup	25	5	3	1	Tr
White beans	1/2 cup	150	28	6	9	1
Yellow beans	1/2 cup	22	5	3	1	Tr
Beef						
Bottom round	3 oz	235	0	0	24	14
Brisket	3 oz	250	0	0	23	17
Chuck blade	3 oz	295	0	0	23	22
Flank steak	3 oz	225	0	0	23	14
Hamburger meat, regular	3 oz	250	0	0	20	18
Pastrami	2 oz	90	2	Tr	12	4
Porterhouse steak	3.5 oz	325	0	0	22	26
Pot roast, chuck	3.5 oz	345	0	0	27	26
Prime ribs	3.5 oz	400	0	0	23	34
Roast beef	3.5 oz	290	0	0	25	20
Sirloin steak	3 oz	220	0	0	24	13
T-bone steak	3.5 oz	310	0	0	23	23
Beets, fresh, cooked, slices	1/2 cup	38	8	2	2	Tr
Blackberries, fresh	1 cup	75	18	8	1	1
Blueberries fresh	1 cup	80	20	4	1	1
Frozen, sugar-sweetened, thawed	1 cup	185	50	5	1	Tr
Bread						
Cracked wheat bread	1 slice	65	12	1	2	1
Croissant, butter flavor, 4"	1	230	26	2	5	12
Egg bread	1 slice	115	19	1	4	2
English muffin, regular	1 whole	135	26	2	4	1
English muffin, cinnamon/raisin	1 whole	140	28	2	4	2

	SERVING SIZE	CALORIES	TOTAL CARBS (g)	FIBER (g)	PROTEIN (g)	FAT (g)
French bread	1 slice	70	13	1	2	1
Garlic bread	1 slice	150	16	1	3	8
Italian bread	1 slice	65	12	1	2	1
Multigrain bread	1 slice	65	12	2	3	1
Oat/oatmeal bread	1 slice	73	13	1	2	1
Pita bread, 4" pita	1 whole	77	16	1	3	Tr
White bread	1 slice	65	12	1	2	1
White or wheat, light bread	1 slice	45	10	2	2	Tr
Breakfast Sandwich, bacon, egg and cheese on English muffin	1 avg. serving	370	19	2	15	28
Broccoli Fresh, raw, chopped, or diced	1 cup	25	5	3	3	Tr
Brownie, 2" square without frosting	1 square	140	20	1	2	6
Burrito, bean and cheese	1	275	25	2	10	15
Butter, regular, salted or unsalted	1 tbsp	100	Tr	0	Tr	12
Caesar Salad	4 oz	200	7	2	7	17
Cake						
Carrot cake, cream cheese icing	1 piece	485	52	2	5	29
Cheesecake, 1/6 of 17 oz cake	1 piece	260	20	Tr	5	18
Chocolate Cake w/frosting	1 piece	390	70	2	5	13
Coffee Crumb Cake, 2.2 oz	1 piece	265	29	1	4	15
Yellow cake, w/frosting	1 piece	390	70	1	5	12
Cantaloupe, fresh, wedge 1/8 melon	1 wedge	25	6	1	1	Tr
Carrot, fresh, raw, whole, 7" long	1	32	7	2	1	Tr
Cereal						
All-Bran	1 cup	80	23	10	4	1
Cheerios, regular	1 cup	110	23	3	3	2

	SERVING SIZE	CALORIES	TOTAL CARBS (g)	FIBER (g)	PROTEIN (g)	FAT (g)
Raisin Bran	1 cup	180	45	7	1	1
Cereal bar, plain	1 bar	135	28	1	2	2
Fruit filled	1 bar	145	29	1	2	2
Cheese						
American, pasteurized, regular	1 oz	105	1	0	6	9
Cheddar cheese	1" cube	68	Tr	0	4	6
Cottage cheese, large curd	1 cup	233	6	0	28	10
Cottage cheese, lowfat, 1% fat	1 cup	164	6	0	28	2
Cream cheese, regular cream	1 oz	100	1	0	2	10
lowfat/light	1 tbsp	35	1	0	2	3
fat-free	1 tbsp	15	1	0	2	0
Feta cheese	1 oz	75	1	0	4	6
Chicken, fried						
1/2 breast, about 5 oz meat	1/2 breast	365	13	Tr	35	18
Drumstick, avg. size	1	195	6	Tr	16	11
Thigh, avg. size	1	240	8	Tr	19	14
Wing, avg. size	1	160	5	Tr	10	11
Chicken, roasted or broiled						
1/2 breast, about 3.5 oz meat	1/2 breast	165	0	0	32	4
Drumstick, avg. size	1	75	0	0	12	2
Thigh, avg. size	1	110	0	0	13	6
White meat w/skin	3.5 oz	280	0	0	33	12
Wings, Buffalo, hot	3	210	3	0	22	12
Chocolate						
Hershey's Chocolate bar plain, 1.5 oz bar	1 bar	230	25	1	3	13
Hershey's Nugget, 10g	1 bar	52	6	Tr	1	3

	SERVING SIZE	CALORIES	TOTAL CARBS (g)	FIBER (g)	PROTEIN (g)	FAT (g)
Hershey's Chocolate Kiss	4	102	11	Tr	1	6
Chocolate chip cookie, regular	1	80	12	1	2	3
Crab cake, w/egg, fried	1 cake	95	1	0	12	5
Eggs						
Egg, hard boiled, whole	1	75	1	0	6	5
Egg omelet, plain, milk added	1	105	1	0	7	8
Egg scrambled w/margarine and milk	1	100	1	0	7	7
Eggplant Parmagiana	1/2 cup	265	26	3	6	16
Fish						
Fish fillet, breaded, fried	3 oz	190	17	1	10	9
Fish sandwich, 3 oz. fried fish fillet	1 avg.					
with tartar sauce and cheese	serving	530	48	Tr	22	29
Orange roughy, baked or broiled	3 oz	75	0	0	16	1
Salmon, baked or broiled	3 oz	185	0	0	23	9
canned, pink	3 oz	118	0	0	17	5
Shrimp, breaded, fried	2 large	110	5	Tr	10	6
Sole, breaded, fried fillet	3 oz	190	17	1	13	8
Trout, baked or broiled	3 oz	145	0	0	21	6
Tuna, baked or broiled	3 oz	120	0	0	25	1
Flour, all-purpose flour, white	1 cup	455	95	3	13	1
Whole wheat flour	1 cup	407	87	15	16	2
French fries, thin, shoestring strips, 3 oz	20 fries	130	22	2	2	4
Restaurant type, regular fries	1 med	350	48	5	5	15
French toast	2 slices	250	38	1	8	8
Grapefruit, pink, red,						
or white fresh, 3 3/4" diameter	1	80	18	3	2	Tr

	SERVING SIZE	CALORIES	TOTAL CARBS (g)	FIBER (g)	PROTEIN (g)	FAT (g)
Grapes, fresh, medium size, all types	10 grapes	35	9	1	Tr	Tr
Ham, lean, roasted	3 oz	130	1	0	16	7
Regular	2 slices	150	3	0	21	5
Hamburger, 4 oz burger w/o cheese	1	420	37	2	23	20
Hot dog on bun w/ catsup and mustard	1 avg. serving	245	19	1	10	15
Ice cream, chocolate regular	1/2 cup	145	19	1	3	7
Vanilla ice cream regular	1/2 cup	135	16	0	2	7
Lentil, cooked	1/2 cup	115	20	8	9	1
Lettuce, loose leaf pieces, shredded or chopped	1 cup	10	2	1	1	Tr
Macaroni and cheese	1 cup	300	40	3	10	10
Mayonnaise, regular	1 tbsp	100	Tr	0	Tr	11
Fat-free	1 tbsp	10	2	0	Tr	0
Light	1 tbsp	50	1	0	Tr	5
Meatless burger						
Single patty, broiled	1 patty	100	9	4	15	1
Cooked, crumbled	1 cup	230	7	5	22	13
Muffin, avg size, 2 1/2" diameter,	1 serving	160	28	2	3	4
Bran w/raisins	1 serving	175	36	4	4	5
Mushroom, fresh, raw, slices	1 cup	18	3	1	2	Tr
Nuts, whole almonds, about 24	1 oz	165	6	3	6	14
Peanuts, dry roasted, about 20 nuts	1 oz	168	7	3	5	15
Pecans, 10 whole or 20 halves	1 oz	195	4	3	3	20
Walnuts, 7 whole	1 oz	185	4	2	4	18
Oatmeal, plain, sweetened	1/2 cup	75	13	2	3	1
Fruit-flavored	1 pkt	135	26	2	3	2

	SERVING SIZE	CALORIES	TOTAL CARBS (g)	FIBER (g)	PROTEIN (g)	FAT (g)
Oil, olive	1 tbsp	119	0	0	0	14
Oil, vegetable	1 tbsp	120	0	0	0	14
Onion, fresh, raw, 2 1/2" diameter	1 whole	42	9	2	1	Tr
Orange, fresh, medium size, 3" diameter	1	70	15	3	1	Tr
Pancake, 4" diameter. Regular, toaster type	1	82	16	1	2	1
Regular, from mix or scratch	1	90	17	1	2	2
Pasta Alfredo Primavera	1 cup	280	44	3	11	7
Pasta salad w/dressing	1 cup	250	32	2	5	10
Peach, fresh, whole, medium size, 2 1/2" diameter	1	42	11	2	1	Tr
Peanut butter regular, smooth	1 tbsp	95	3	1	4	8
Regular, chunky	1 tbsp	95	3	1	4	8
Pear, fresh, 2" diameter.	1	50	13	4	1	Tr
Peas, green	1/2 cup	60	11	4	4	Tr
Lentils	1/2 cup	115	20	8	9	1
Navy peas	1/2 cup	125	24	6	8	1
Peas and carrots	1/2 cup	40	8	3	3	Tr
Pineapple, fresh, diced or sliced	1 cup	76	19	2	1	1
Pizza, 1/8 of 12" pizza, cheese	1 slice	140	21	1	8	3
Pepperoni and cheese	1 slice	180	20	1	10	7
Pizza, Pan						
Cheese	1 slice	270	39	1	15	6
Pepperoni and cheese	1 slice	310	39	1	19	8
One meat w/vegetables	1 slice	320	38	2	15	12
Three meat w/vegetables	1 slice	405	40	2	24	17
Pizza, stuffed crust						
Pepperoni and cheese	1 slice	350	39	1	20	14

	SERVING SIZE	CALORIES	TOTAL CARBS (g)	FIBER (g)	PROTEIN (g)	FAT (g)
Three meat w/vegetables	1 slice	450	40	2	21	21
Pizza rolls, 1'', frozen, heated						
with cheese and one meat	5 pieces	175	20	1	9	7
Plantain, without peel						
Fresh, medium size	1	218	57	4	2	1
Cooked, slices	1 cup	180	48	4	1	Tr
Plum						
Fresh, whole, medium, 2'' diameter	1	36	9	1	1	Tr
Canned, in heavy syrup	1 cup	230	60	3	1	Tr
Canned, in juice	1 cup	146	38	3	1	Tr
Pomegranate, avg size, raw	1	105	26	2	2	1
Popcorn						
Air popped	1 cup	30	6	1	1	Tr
Caramel coated w/peanuts	1 cup	170	34	2	3	3
Caramel coated w/o peanuts	1 cup	150	28	2	1	5
Cheese flavored	1 cup	60	6	1	1	4
Microwave, butter flavor	1 cup	40	4	1	1	2
Microwave, butter, reduced fat	1 cup	30	5	1	1	1
Popped in oil	1 cup	55	6	1	1	3
Popped in oil, buttered	1 cup	75	6	1	1	5
Popcorn cake, plain	1	38	8	Tr	1	Tr
Butter flavor	1	40	8	Tr	1	Tr
Carmel	1	48	11	Tr	1	Tr
Poppyseed pastry filling	1 tbsp	65	14	1	1	1
Pork (weights for meat w/o bones)						
Bacon, regular	3 slices	110	Tr	0	6	9

	SERVING SIZE	CALORIES	TOTAL CARBS (g)	FIBER (g)	PROTEIN (g)	FAT (g)
Bacon, Canadian	3 slices	125	1	0	17	6
Boston butt, roasted, lean	3 oz	205	0	0	27	9
Picnic pork	3.5 oz	280	Tr	0	20	21
Pork chop, loin cut						
broiled, lean and fat	3 oz	205	0	0	24	11
broiled, lean only	3 oz	170	0	0	26	7
pan fried, lean and fat	3 oz	235	0	0	25	14
pan fried, lean only	3 oz	195	0	0	27	9
Rib Roast, lean and fat	3 oz	215	0	0	23	13
lean only	3 oz	195	0	0	24	9
Sausage						
breakfast link, small	1 link	70	Tr	0	3	6
breakfast patty, small	1 patty	80	Tr	0	3	7
sausage, regular	2 oz	120	1	0	7	10
sausage, lowfat	2 oz	80	6	0	7	2
Polish Kielbasa sausage	2 oz	120	Tr	0	8	10
Vienna sausage, 2" links	2 links	90	Tr	0	4	8
Shoulder cut, braised, lean and fat	3 oz	280	0	0	24	20
lean only	3 oz	210	0	0	27	10
Potato, baked, medium size w/skin	1	220	51	5	5	Tr
Hash-browned potatoes	1 cup	280	32	2	4	14
Mashed, w/milk and margarine	1 cup	220	35	4	4	9
Potato chips, plain, regular	1 oz	155	15	1	2	10
Fat-free chips	1 oz	75	17	1	2	Tr
Potato salad	1 cup	360	28	3	7	21
Pretzels sticks, regular	25	58	12	1	1	1

	SERVING SIZE	CALORIES	TOTAL CARBS (g)	FIBER (g)	PROTEIN (g)	FAT (g)
Pudding chocolate, regular	1/2 cup	150	25	1	3	5
Sugar-free	1/2 cup	110	18	1	2	1
Raisins, golden or natural, not packed	1 cup	435	115	6	5	1
Raspberries, fresh	1 cup	60	14	8	1	1
Ravioli, beef	1 cup	255	44	1	12	4
Cheese	1 cup	265	44	1	11	5
Rice dishes, plain, brown long grain, prep. w/butter	1 cup	315	45	4	5	13
Rice, flavored w/beef or pork	1 cup	280	52	3	8	4
Rice, fried w/shrimp	1 cup	260	44	3	9	5
Rice fried w/vegetables	1 cup	255	48	3	7	4
Salad, tossed						
All vegetable salad, no dressing	1 1/2 cups	60	11	4	3	Tr
w/regular dressing, any type	1 1/2 cups	200	6	1	10	17
Sandwich, w/2.5 oz. meat	1	455	51	2	22	19
Tuna salad w/mayo, lettuce	1	585	55	2	30	28
Seeds, pumpkin seeds, roasted	1 oz	148	4	1	9	12
Sunflower seeds, dry roasted	1 oz	165	7	3	5	14
Soup						
Chicken noodle, regular	1 cup	75	9	1	4	2
Chicken noodle, chunky	1 cup	175	17	4	13	6
Clam chowder, New England	1 cup	165	17	2	9	7
Cream of chicken soup, prep w/water	1 cup	117	9	Tr	3	7
Lentil soup, low-fat	1 cup	125	20	6	8	2
Minestrone	1 cup	85	11	1	4	3
Onion soup	1 cup	100	19	4	4	2
Pea soup	1 cup	160	26	3	9	3

	SERVING SIZE	CALORIES	TOTAL CARBS (g)	FIBER (g)	PROTEIN (g)	FAT (g)
Tomato soup, prep w/water	1 cup	85	17	1	2	2
Vegetable soup	1 cup	72	12	1	2	2
Vegetable beef soup	1 cup	90	11	1	7	2
Sour cream, regular	1 tbsp	25	1	0	Tr	3
Fat-free	1 tbsp	12	2	0	Tr	0
Soy burger, broiled	1 patty	100	9	3	15	1
Spaghetti						
Plain, cooked	1 cup	195	40	2	7	1
w/meatballs in tomato sauce	1 cup	240	41	3	7	4
Spinach, frozen, chopped, cooked	1 cup	53	10	6	6	Tr
Strawberries, fresh, medium size	10	40	9	3	1	Tr
Sugar	1 tbsp	45	12	0	0	0
Restaurant-size packet	1 pkt	24	6	0	0	0
Brown sugar, packed, one cup	1 cup	827	214	0	0	0
Sweet potato baked w/skin 4" x 2"	1 whole	165	38	4	3	Tr
Tangerine, fresh, med, 2" diameter	1	37	9	2	1	Tr
Tater Tots fried potatoes	10	175	24	3	3	8
Tofu, plain, cooked, 4 oz	1/2 cup	80	2	Tr	9	4
Tomato, fresh, raw, avg. size 2" diameter	1 whole	26	6	1	1	Tr
Fresh, raw, cherry tomato	1 whole	4	1	Tr	Tr	Tr
Fresh, slices	1 slice	4	1	Tr	Tr	Tr
Tomato sauce	1 cup	74	18	3	3	Tr
Tortellini, cheese filling	1 cup	270	40	2	12	7
Meat filling	1 cup	340	55	1	21	9
Tortilla chips, regular	1 oz	140	18	2	2	7
Lowfat, baked	1 oz	115	22	2	4	1

	SERVING SIZE	CALORIES	TOTAL CARBS (g)	FIBER (g)	PROTEIN (g)	FAT (g)
Tuna salad, w/tuna in oil, mayo, and dressing	$1/_2$ cup	190	9	0	16	10
Turkey, roast						
Light and dark meat	3 oz	145	3	0	22	5
Light meat only	3 oz	135	0	0	25	4
Dark meat only	3 oz	160	0	0	25	6
Veal						
Chop, loin, braised	3.5 oz	285	0	0	30	17
Cutlet, braised, lean and fat	3 oz	180	0	0	31	5
Vegetable burger, broiled	1 patty	100	9	4	15	1
Yogurt						
Vanilla, regular	$1/_2$ cup	120	18	0	3	4
Vanilla, fat-free	$1/_2$ cup	110	23	0	4	0
Made w/skim milk	$1/_2$ cup	120	15	0	13	0
Fruit, regular varieties	$1/_2$ cup	135	20	1	5	3
Fruit flavor, sugar-free	$1/_2$ cup	95	16	0	9	Tr

Calories Burned During Activity and Exercise (per hour)

ACTIVITY	125 lbs	150 lbs	175 lbs	200 lbs
			PERSON'S WEIGHT	
Aerobics: high impact	420	504	588	672
Aerobics: low impact	330	396	462	528
Bicycling: > 20 mph	990	1188	1386	1584
Bicycling: 12.-13.9 mph	480	576	672	768
Bicycling: 14-15.9 mph	600	720	840	960
Bicycling: 16-19 mph	720	864	1008	1152
Bowling	180	216	252	288
Circuit Training	480	576	672	768
Cross-Country Skiing	480	576	672	768
Dancing	360	432	504	576
Downhill Skiing	360	432	504	576
Elliptical Trainer	540	648	756	864
Gardening	270	324	378	432
Golf: carrying clubs	330	396	462	528
Golf: using cart	210	252	294	336
Hiking: cross-country	360	432	504	576
Ice Skating	420	504	588	672
Martial Arts	540	648	756	864
Mowing the Lawn (hand)	330	396	462	528
Racquetball: casual	420	504	588	672
Raking Leaves	240	288	336	384
Rollerblading	529	604	746	820

ACTIVITY	PERSON'S WEIGHT			
	125 lbs	150 lbs	175 lbs	200 lbs
Rope Jumping	600	704	840	960
Running: 12 min/mile	480	576	672	768
Running: 10 min/mile	600	720	840	960
Sitting	68	81	95	108
Sleeping	38	45	53	60
Stationary Bicycling	420	504	588	672
Step Aerobics, High-Impact	600	720	840	960
Step Aerobics, Low-Impact	420	504	588	672
Swimming	600	720	840	960
Tennis	420	505	588	672
Walk/Jog	360	432	504	576
Walk: 17 min/mile	240	288	336	384
Walk: 15 min/mile	270	324	378	432
Water Aerobics	240	288	336	462

Progress Chart

Week	Weight	Chest	Waist	Hips
	START			
1 2-8 Jan	81.5			
2 9-15 Jan				
3				
4				
5				
6				
7				
8				
9				
10				
11				
12				
TOTALS				